Fight Memory Loss with Art

Learn an Art or Craft to delay dementia and Alzheimer's, Take up drawing, painting, sculpture, music or another language to keep your brain healthy

Tim Vincent

Disclaimer and Terms of Use: The Author and Publisher has strived to be as accurate and complete as possible in the creation of this book, notwithstanding the fact that he does not warrant or represent at any time that the contents within are accurate due to the rapidly changing nature of science and medicine. While all attempts have been made to verify information provided in this publication, the Author and Publisher assumes no responsibility for errors, omissions, or contrary interpretation of the subject matter herein. Any perceived slights of specific persons, peoples, or organizations are unintentional. In practical advice books, like anything else in life, there are no guarantees of any results obtained. Readers are cautioned to rely on their own judgment and seek professional medical advice about their individual circumstances and to act accordingly.

First Printing, 2015

ISBN - 13: 978-1517711986

ISBN - 10: 1517711983

Printed in the United States of America

Dedication

For Alan and Chris who helped with the art photos

Fight Memory Loss with Art

Learn an Art or Craft to delay dementia and Alzheimer's, Take up drawing, painting, sculpture, music or another language to keep your brain healthy

Table of Contents

Introduction

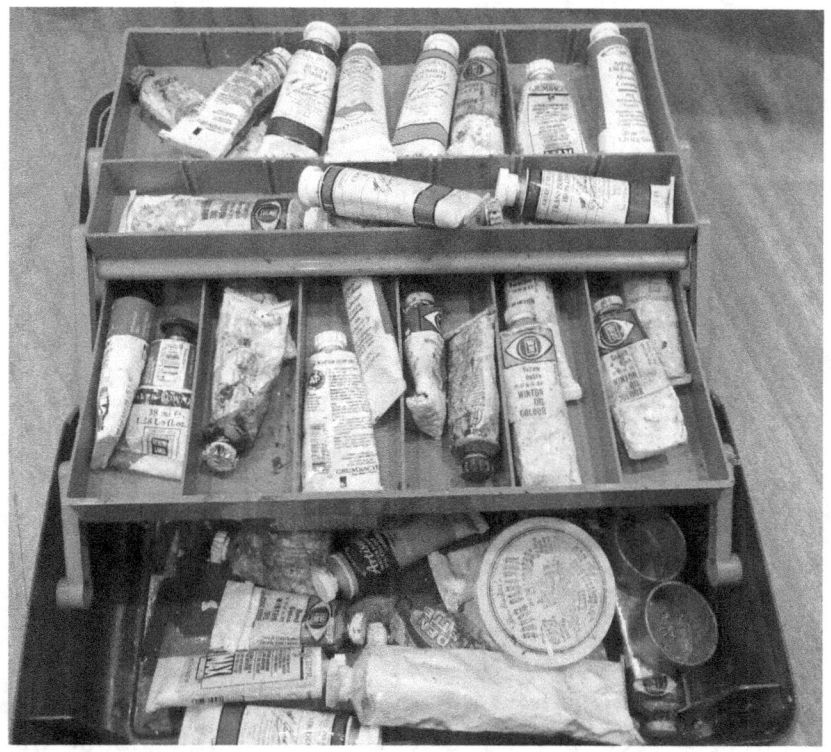

One of the greatest worries that people have as they get older is that they will suffer from a brain wasting disease such as Alzheimer's or other forms of dementia. This can be particularly worrying if somebody in your near family has suffered from it and you have seen the devastating effects of these conditions for yourself. My mother suffered from dementia and I saw her turn from an articulate lively individual into a person who just didn't do anything and couldn't even recognise me. These situations make you worry about your own future. It certainly made me think about what was going to happen to me. There are some sensible things that everybody should do in terms of their general health in order to avoid the risk of dementia and these consist of: not smoking, or giving it up if you currently smoke; keeping your weight under control and avoiding foods that might lead to diabetes. Despite these reasonable medical suggestions, there is a lack of understanding as to what can be done to actually promote good brain or mental health and the things that can help to put off the inevitable decline in brain function due to ageing.

It is interesting to note that not all people are affected by dementia and that started me thinking about why certain people seem to be more susceptible to the condition. With other parts of the body we often say that you 'need to use it, or you will lose it'. This certainly seems to ring true when you consider other age related conditions such as some forms of arthritis. A few years ago I suffered with arthritis in my knee and had got to the point of having to use a walking stick. After some physiotherapy to relieve the condition, I took up an idea that I had found out, about trying to walk 6000 steps a day. Since making this decision and using a pedometer app on my phone I have managed to keep the pain of arthritis in my knee at bay. It is still there but the 6000 steps are enough to keep the knee joint lubricated and stop the pain returning. A number of people have said the same thing about the functioning of the brain. There have indeed been some much publicised 'brain training' schemes which are designed to keep your mental activity honed. These all involve making your brain solve novel problems. There are computer apps that keep a record of your scores and you, in sense, compete against yourself to get better at solving the problems. This would all seem to make sense: keep using your brain and you will remain lucid for longer. There has been some success with these schemes and people have reported benefits from their brain training activities. The only problem with this kind of solution is that it has a rather narrow focus. Yes, you get better at solving the set problems, but this isn't all that the brain is about.

There are many different areas of the brain that do very specific things. For a healthy brain these different brain areas have to work together. A scheme for maintaining overall brain activity can't be a 'one trick pony' because it has to offer stimulation to many areas of the brain at the same time and encourage them to interact. This is where Art comes into the frame. You may wonder why something like art could possibly be as important as this. In general life art just doesn't seem that important to us. However, as young children, drawing and painting are the activities that we love to do and perhaps as adults we lose our respect for it.

To get an idea of the importance of art to the human condition you have to look a little more towards our origins. Indeed, on the path towards our modern age art has been very important. Over the centuries creating art has inspired, comforted and energised us by seizing our imagination. Art has a definite power over us and gives perception about what it is to be a part of the human species. For it to have lasted so long there must be something important about it. In fact, if you look back in time, you find that there has never been a culture without its own forms of art whether that be drawing, painting, music or poetry. Art must be giving us something that is fundamental to the human condition.

Back in the day when man was a hunter gatherer, even though most of his effort was spent just trying to survive, time was still found for art whether that be cave paintings, dance or music. Art must have therefore been very important to them and that importance probably had something to do with health. It is possible, that since the modern use of pills for all our ills we have forgotten about all these art inspired things that helped us along our way. Perhaps it is time to rediscover the value of art in maintaining a healthy human person.

How Memory Works

Having some understanding about what we can and can't expect from our memory can help us to work out what can be done to improve it and in turn protect us against dementia and related conditions. Over the years, scientists and the general public have struggled to understand the workings of the brain and as a result a lot of miss information has entered the public domain and distorted the way memory conditions have been treated. A lot of methods of memory improvement have been sold to the public based on this miss information. It therefore pays to know about those methods that simply don't work and never will work.

We tend to think that memories are set in stone once you have them. A bit like a digital recording you might make on your mobile phone. However, it seems that memories aren't as predictable as we would like to think. Believe it or not, your memories can be changed by the things around you that you are interacting with. These could be as mundane as the reasons you are remembering, your feelings at the time, external interactions such as smells and familiar objects or people, and even the number of times that you access that particular memory. So rather than being like a video film, they are more like a story that somebody is telling you.

Through the use of computers we have gotten used to the idea that memories are stored in a particular location on a particular memory device such as a hard drive. We seem to have decided that the brain remembers things in a similar way. It seems, however, that memories are scattered about the brain in different locations and when we try to remember something the memory has to be put together again from all these different pieces in what you might say is like a jigsaw.

The amount of memory space and working space of the brain isn't set out from the start. The brain can change in size and grow by adding new nerve cells and nerve pathways. The more you ask of your brain the more that it will change and give you the functioning power that you want. Making your brain work hard is a good way to make sure that it stays healthy and able to deal with all that life throws at you. Although we do lose a certain number of brain cells as we age this is a normal process. We can cause the brain to add more by simply giving it some 'brain exercise'.

If we want to give our brain some exercise we tend to think about doing something that seems difficult such as crosswords or playing brain training games. The problem here is that although the tasks are difficult they are all rather similar and the whole thing becomes rather too familiar to us. Familiarity doesn't exercise the brain at all. What it really needs are tasks that change and are complicated at the same time. If you concentrate at doing crosswords you just become very good at doing this one task. What you need is something that varies a lot and is complicated to complete.

We have always been told that as you get older your memory gets worse, but this is not always the case. Some 90 year old seniors are still as bright as a pin. Inevitably some memory is lost along the way, but not as much as people think. In actual fact, it seems that young adults are more likely to be forgetful on a daily basis compared to older people. It is thought that defective life style choices are to blame: including the over use of drink, drugs and electronic devices. Lack of sleep and too much stress also play their part in the poor memory of younger people. Many people are trying to do more than one thing at once. This multitasking ability seems very popular these days especially with having to deal with mobile phones, laptops, tablets and the like. Quickly moving from one task to another in this fashion may be trendy, but it isn't very good for our poor brains. The penalty for this is poor attention spans, less ability to learn, low performance and poor short term memory. Attention spans have gotten shorter over the centuries, until we are now in a situation that the average American has an attention span less than a common goldfish! (Not a Joke: scientists have proved it!)

As people get older they tend to worry about ending up with dementia and they often get a heightened awareness of small memory lapses. It is worth considering that everybody gets these kind of glitches no matter how old that they are. How many times have you ended up in a room and wondered why you are there? Everybody experiences this and it is not a sign of dementia creeping up on us. Added to this are other effects of daily life that can affect the performance of our memory. These include stress, lack of sleep, drinking, smoking, low levels of exercise and even certain medications that we may be taking for other health conditions.

Supplements that are advertised as being able to improve your memory are generally bogus. Despite this, many people are duped by the claims made and this is especially the case when older people are already fearful about getting dementia. In addition to not doing the job that they are advertised to do they may also cause side effects that they don't want you to know about. There are also similar tablets sold that students use when trying to swat for exams. These often sharpen alertness and concentration but their effects are relatively short lived and the brain may need time to recover from them after

15

they are used. They certainly aren't for use in the long term and if they are used may cause more harm than good.

One of the recent discoveries is the relationship between physical exercise and brain health. Exercise can help all parts of the body and should be a part of everybody's life. Taking part in exercise improves circulation which distributes oxygen more efficiently around the body including to the brain. Improved circulation has been shown to be good for the brain and leads to better memory, improved ability to learn new things and even the growth of new brain cells. Add to this that exercise can make you feel happier and relieve stress then you are on to a winner as far as helping to protect your brain against dementia type illnesses. Meditation is another thing that has been shown to be good at keeping your brain healthy as well. Meditation can act as a stress buster. Exercise and meditation can be used side by side with the art therapy ideas that are discussed in this book. The three of these together makes sure that you will be on the winning team as far as you brain is concerned.

The Benefits of Art

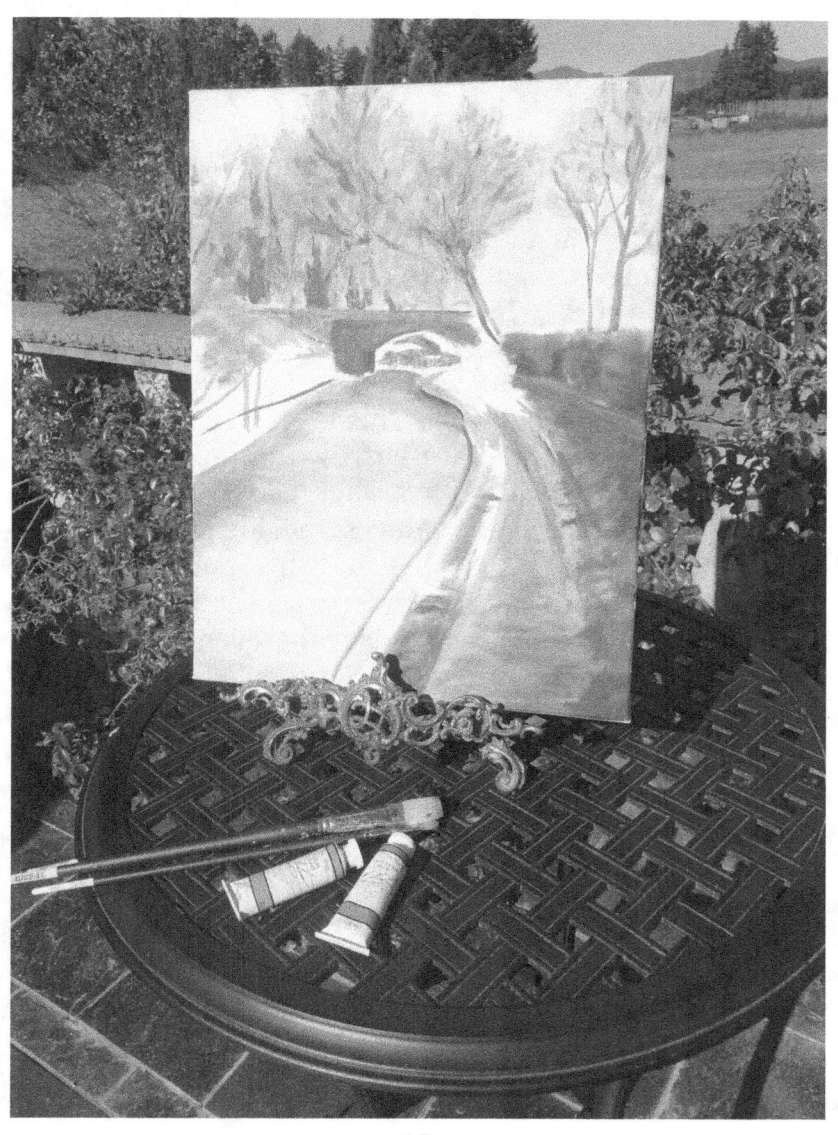

Even just looking at art can have a positive effect on people. In fact viewing art in the form of pictures and paintings is already used in old people's homes with people suffering dementia. This is a form of art therapy and it works because everybody has an opinion about art. People start out by saying whether they like it or not. This can then produce discussions and thinking as to why a particular piece of art is good or not. At first it would appear that viewing art would be a purely passive activity but as can be seen, with discussion it can result in lots of stimulation for the brain.

Whereas viewing art has some benefits, the greatest gains can be obtained from producing art yourself. The creation of art is a great way to keep your brain active. In addition to this, making art is open to anyone. Anybody can start to do art even if they haven't done that much in the past. A lot of people were probably put off art while they were at school. In class you would have noticed that some people were very good at art. This leads to the very wrong idea that certain people are born with a gift for art and that they are the only ones that can be involved in creating art. This then produces the idea that without natural talent there is nothing that the rest of us can do about it. It is fair to say that those with the natural talent may go on to be recognised artists and even earn a living from it, but anybody can start an art based hobby at any time. You can teach yourself using 'how to' style books and videos or even gain proper instruction by joining an art class. With help along the way, even an individual with only a little talent can be encouraged to create their own art. For people who have retired there are often art courses that are available for them to start an interest in making art works. If you have ever thought about doing some art, the extra time gained during retirement is an ideal time to start and perhaps you could even join a course or art group. Libraries and community organisations often have details of what is available and so these are good places to find out what is going on in your area.

In the end, it really is of no consequence whether you think you have any artistic talent or not. You can start out on your artistic journey just because it is enjoyable to do so. You will quickly find that with practice and perhaps some lessons you will find that perhaps you did have some talent but it had become hidden away over the years. Of course, it doesn't hurt to remember that, all of the time you spend enjoying yourself creating art, you will be vitalizing your brain and improving your health and happiness.

The kinds of things that happen once you pick up that brush and start painting are very interesting to consider. Producing a new artistic creation will definitely spark your imagination. Earlier on in the introduction it was indicated that there are different parts of the brain which have particular jobs to do. As well as this, the brain is also divided up into the left and right sides. Each side is associated with its own particular thought patterns. In our journey through life we may tend to use one side of the brain a little more than the other. Those people who use the right side of their brain to a greater extent tend to be more artistic. In these people, doing art later in life will tend to improve the skills that are already there and they will become more creative. People who are more scientific or analytical tend to be more left side of the brain oriented. In this case, starting to do art will help to encourage both imagination and creativity.

When people are producing art they have to look at the things around them in a lot more detail. They become more observant especially when it comes to things like light and dark, colour, shape and position, distances and movement. You have to consider the environment around you and see the detail involved in your art project.

Despite not being analytical in nature art does improve skills in the area of solving problems. An artistic problem is, however, unlikely to have that definitive answer found in physics and mathematics. You have to come up with your own individual answer to the problems you come across and perhaps even try to think the unthinkable.

Producing a piece of art from virtually nothing can give a feeling of great achievement. This will also make you want to show it to other people. In showing others our work we can end up increasing our feelings of confidence and self-respect. These kinds of feedback are important when it comes to our own feelings of wellbeing.

Spending time away from the daily grind of life being artistically creative can help to relieve a lot of stress. Hobbies like this tend to be rather relaxing while you are doing them. The progress that you make through time will also feel rewarding. This relaxation leads to lower stress levels which in turn enhances feelings of wellbeing.

Art helps to improve our thinking abilities including memory and this has been shown to work with people having many different brain conditions. When art therapy is used with people suffering dementia there can be up to a seventy percent achievement in the improvement of their memories. It is believed that a lot of this success is down to increased connections between the left and right sides of the brain.

As well as helping with dementia it has been found that art also helps with a wide range of medical conditions including depression, anxiety, pain, post-traumatic stress disorder, bipolar conditions, high blood pressure and even cancer. In this way art could be considered a kind of medicine in its own right. Sometimes art has been shown to work where nothing else has done so. This is particularly the case with soldiers returning from stressful battle situations.

A new study in the US sheds more light on the effect of arts and crafts on memory difficulties and how they develop as people age. From the Neurology journal it follows two hundred and fifty six people that were in the years eighty five through to eighty nine. None of them had any memory difficulties when the study began and consisted of both women and men. The study collected data over a 4 year period. Data was collected on a number of aspects of their life including how much art related activities that they did. This related to such things as drawing, sculpting and painting as well as the craft based activities of pottery, woodwork, sewing and making quilts. Socialising was also examined and in particular, time with friendship groups, book clubs, bible clubs and travel to different places. They were also asked to account for the amount of time they spent on the internet including purchasing things. At the end of the study they analysed the data and determined how their activities protected them against small losses of thinking and memory ability. This was expressed as a percentage compared to people not doing the activities. Here are the results:

Art activities 73% less prone to problems

Crafts 45% less prone to problems

Computer use 52% less prone to problems

Active social life 55% less prone to problems

Medical problems such as high blood pressure and depression in younger life have also been implicated in promoting memory and thinking problems once people get older. Despite this the results clearly show that art and craft activities can protect against getting memory and thinking problems later in life.

The term 'art therapy' appears to make it sound like you need some kind of therapist to be involved. There are indeed people who are art therapists, but they tend to work with people that have more serious health problems. The professional art therapist will encourage these people to get involved with art and will have specialised programs for the people involved to follow. If you don't have a serious health problem then there is no need to see an art therapist at all. The main thing is to get yourself involved in an art project. Perhaps you might decide to take up painting. In this case, it would be sufficient for you to do your painting hobby a few times each week. Once you are involved in your art, it is of course therapy and no professional art therapist has been involved at all. Sometimes the first step into this new world is the hardest. There are lots of prejudices that we carry around with us and as a result you may find yourself thinking that art is only for artists and that it isn't really worth bothering with. This is a big mistake because art is actually a part of us all. Art is for all of us and inside each individual lies a flicker of creativity hidden away.

All of us have our 'when I have the time' lists of things that we would someday like to do. You might have always fancied the idea of painting, sculpting or drawing but never got round to it. Maybe sculpting or playing a musical instrument is one of the ideas that you put away for a rainy day. Whatever your desire, now is the time to do something about it especially now that the benefits of such activities are becoming so apparent.

Helping Friends and Relatives with Art Therapy

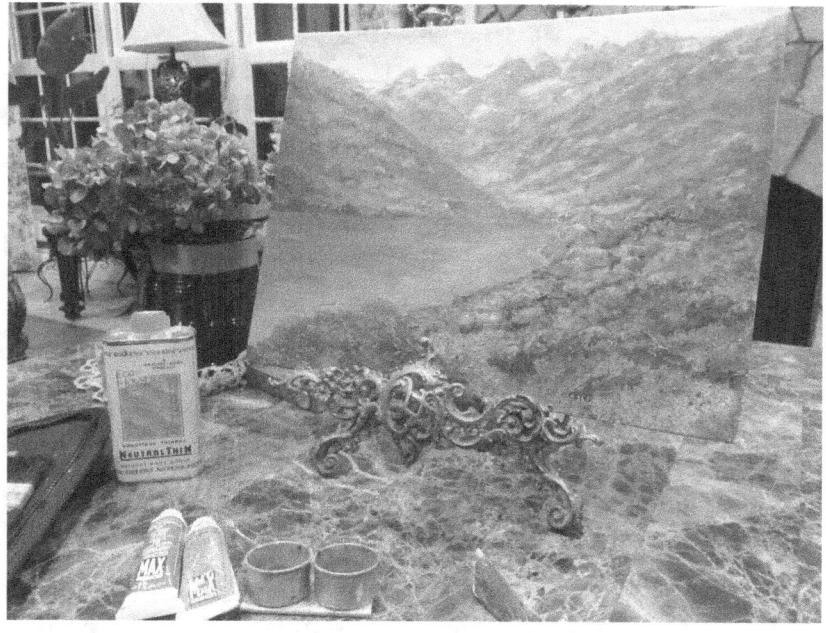

If you have a friend or relative that suffers from dementia you can help them by encouraging them to do some art activities. Depending on how badly they are affected you can come up with some suitable things for them to do. Art therapy produces a rich background and context that will stimulate the imagination of people suffering from dementia. Art therapy becomes more important in the later stages of the condition where individuals may have lost talking and conversational skills. In the form of a pleasant activity it can give a different way for people to communicate with others. Individuals doing art feel more at home with themselves and less under pressure. As well as allowing them to express themselves it can help them to get some of their old motor skills back, such as using finger and hands, so that they can do more things in general.

In a family situation art activities give a new way for them to communicate especially if using words has become very difficult. It can help to bring families together as well as allowing younger children to appreciate their elderly relatives who, with this condition, may have become somewhat distant or frightening. The dementia sufferers themselves may find that joining in helps them to relax so that problem behaviours become less pronounced.

The sorts of art activities that are used have to be simple enough to be completed so that the dementia sufferer gets some sense of achievement in the end. Painting and sculpting are ideal choices in this respect.

The best way to start off a session is to suggest drawing or painting a family situation from the past. This may allow them to recall things from their childhood which will allow them to start drawing such things as the old family home, a place they went on holiday or other more easily remembered things.

There are safety issues to be considered and as a result it is best to make sure that the materials used are of a nontoxic nature, in case they get swallowed during the activity. Labels on paints, glues and so on should be checked before use. You can, of course, make your own paints and clay for sculpting and in that way ensure that the materials are completely safe by using only ingredients that can be eaten. The materials that are used are best if they are brightly coloured. In this way they tend to be more stimulating for dementia sufferers to use.

Including some interesting things such as bright card, coloured boxes, string, old pictures and cloth material can also help with developing the imagination And producing artistic ideas.

Relaxation is a key to success and therefore you should ensure that the environment is nice and pleasant. This can be done by providing warm lighting and calming music as a backdrop to the activity. As well as selecting activities that can be reasonably easily achieved it may also be necessary to chivvy them along a little with encouraging comments as they work. Such things as 'nice work', 'great attempt' and 'I like that' go a long way to keeping them on track. As they work you can talk to them about particular aspects such as the colours used and shapes that they like. If the person is still articulate to some degree they may be able to respond to general questions about the art they have created and allow for conversations to be instigated.

Once completed it is a nice idea to put the items in a gallery that can be viewed later. This gallery doesn't have to be anything special but rather just a wall in the hallway or a noticeboard in the kitchen. This will then allow for the items to be discussed later on and conversations to develop about past events and general interests. All of this will allow for past memories to be retrieved and for socialising in the family. It can also go some way to restoring a sense of worth and pride to a dementia sufferer.

Getting Started in Art

There are a number of ideas that you might like to think about when it comes to taking up a form of art. There are great benefits to be obtained from going to an organised class. These benefits are greater than just the art itself because you will be going somewhere different, having to keep to a class time, mixing with other likeminded people and have to keep to a schedule of producing art work or doing homework tasks. All of these benefits and more are discussed in the subsections below.

Despite the benefits of going to an art class it might not be suitable for you. Everybody is different and everybody's personal situation is also different. For this reason a more 'do it yourself' option may be preferable. If you have a friend who is also into art or wants to get into art, then working together could be a good option. In this way you can support each other and 'jolly each other along' on the way. Talking to a likeminded individual is also a good thing and has benefits on the communication front. If you have a friend who is good at art you might ask them if they would mentor you and give advice on what to do and see how well you are progressing.

As for DIY lessons there are a number of resources from online courses, YouTube videos to physical books. Books themselves don't have to be expensive. Local libraries often have good sections on arts and crafts and so you could find suitable books to borrow. Charity book stores and stalls also often have a good selection of art instruction books.

The main problem with a DIY approach is keeping up your efforts. Without other people reminding you to do your art projects they can slip from your mind or be put off to another day due to other household tasks. However, once you get into an art project it can become so enjoyable that it is difficult to put down. This is a good thing, as you will have the art bug and it will become one of your regular hobbies. To prevent getting isolated with your work you could show relatives and friends what you are doing, especially if you have a finished piece of artwork that you are proud of. If you have the space in your home it is nice to put aside a part of it for your art activities. Something like a spare room or a corner of the garage is ideal. In this way you can leave your art equipment and art project ready set up for you to continue working when you need or want to. There nothing more off-putting than having to keep putting equipment away after use and having to drag it out each time you want to use it. Sometimes this can become a barrier in itself to getting on with the art and it can be an excuse to procrastinate or just plain do nothing. I like to have my project at hand so that I can just disappear for an hour or so and do a little more. When things are easy to pick up and start you can easily slot in even a few sessions of work at different times during the day.

Going to an Art Class

In a study undertaken by Newcastle University in the UK a number of people were asked to undertake activities that could possibly stimulate brain activity and thus keep it healthy. Tests were done to establish the current brain activities of the volunteers. They were divided into 3 groups and asked to do a particular activity for 8 weeks. One group was asked to do vigorous walking and exercise, another was asked to some popular puzzles including crosswords. The final group was asked to attend an organised art class. The most popular activity was the art class. People were less positive in their reaction to the exercise and puzzle solving groups. At the end of the 8 weeks each person was retested and the differences in mental activity were noted. It was found that all of the groups had improved to some extent but by far the outright winners were the people in the art class group.

It is thought that the art class was more stimulating because it encouraged the people to learn something new. The brain reacts to learning the new skills and becomes more active. It didn't matter how old you were or how much art you had done previously. Art such as drawing and painting has extra rewards compared to the other tasks because it also involves getting the muscles controlling your hands to do the right things at the right times. Other factors that were considered in this mini study included the benefits of standing rather than sitting. The artists often spent long times standing at an easel doing their paintings. It has become known that standing helps to keep people healthy. Not only does it burn up more energy than sitting it also helps to keep the digestive system healthy preventing debilitating conditions such as diverticulosis and bowel cancer developing. It also appears that maintaining a social life is important for keeping your brain active. The art group met up on a regular basis even outside of the normal class times. Socialising like this allows for more discussion and conversation which in turn helps to keep your mind active. It is a sad fact that the older we get the more cut off from the rest of the world that we become. Without work and friends to meet we become isolated and more inward looking. This situation isn't good for keeping your brain working.

Attending an art class therefore has many benefits for brain health and also the general health of the rest of your body. This doesn't mean to say that it has to be a traditional art class that is attended. It could equally be any other types of class where you learn new things, keep active in some way and promotes social activity. Perhaps joining a photographic class might be equally as good a choice.

Drawing

Drawing is a good place to start with art. It seems that the need to draw is already with us when we are born. We have a drive to learn how to draw from when we are very young. Other skills like reading, writing and maths have to be taught, but not drawing. Drawing somehow seems to be needed as part of the growing process. Toddlers learn to draw even before they start school. Even from a young age drawing helps us in our everyday lives. Drawings help us to work out what we are thinking and through it we get smarter. How many of us have drawn sketches of things that we wish to make? Through these drawings we can work out what the thing will actually look like and whether it will do its intended job in the end. Drawings have been used by inventors to visualise new ideas and to improve old ones.

Drawing can help you become more self-assured and realise that making mistakes is not always a problem. In a drawing it is easy to put right a mistake and sometimes these mistakes help us to come up with new concepts. Once you start creating your own images you will always be trying to come up with new ways to do your drawings. This is the stuff that helps create those new nerve pathways in the brain and in turn for us to get wiser and sharper.

During the drawing process you will start to notice things in more detail. You will tend to remember more about an object or scene after you have drawn it. When something that you are drawing is quite complex such as an insect you will start to recognise all of the parts that it is made up of. You will then quickly learn all of the parts that make up the insect because it is important for getting your drawing right.

Drawings are important. They are often clearer than written or spoken language and help us to remember

31

things too. They can help us to explain things and to follow instructions. Drawings can help us to put over a story or even a joke. They can be subtly changed to get over a point or draw our attention to a particular situation. Just think about political cartoons in our newspapers. Important signs often use drawings to draw our attention to a particular danger or important feature. Just think what it would be like having to read every road sign instead of just glancing at the illustration on the sign. Drawings can be used to make things look more sensational and a good drawing can bring out emotions within us when we look at it.

Within drawings you can articulate feelings, moods and show what we dream about such that they can be communicated to all that view them. In this way drawing is the same as other art forms such as music where emotion is an obvious and important part of each work of art.

You don't need that much equipment to start drawing. You can draw in black and white or in colour. Here are some of the things that you will find most useful in the beginning before you learn what is right for you. They can all be obtained from local art stores or from online shops too.

Some good, soft graphite pencils for drawing. These include HB, 6B, 4B and 2B grades

A pack of high quality coloured pencils

Durable sketchpad

A variety of eraser types such as Pink Pearl, Gum, vinyl and kneaded

Some blending stumps

Quality white and coloured drawing paper of a size 11 inch by 14 inch or larger

Compressed charcoal

Vine charcoal

Chalk pastels

Oil pastels

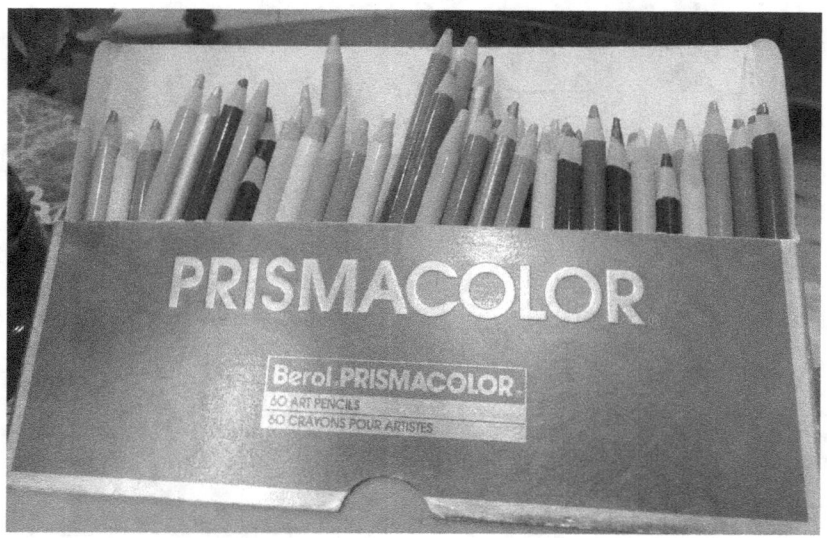

Coloured Art Pencils

In addition to this a large drawing easel that will allow you to stand while you work will also be of benefit. This is because when it comes to keeping fit, standing uses a lot more calories than sitting while you work.

Painting

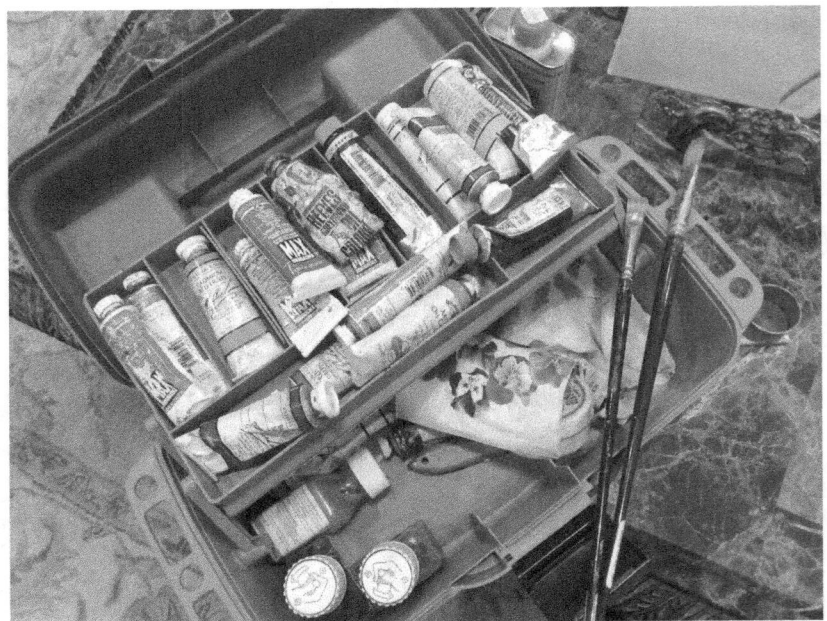

There are lots of thoughts about painting and art: from it being just like keeping a diary to the idea that painting is easy when you don't actually know how to do it. These have all been ways to encourage the new artist into painting. It clearly hasn't really worked because the multitude haven't picked up their brushes and homes aren't filled with palettes and easels. Never the less it is possible to take up painting without all of the commitment to art classes at a college or night school.

One of the best ways to get into the world of painting is to try and do painting every day. This isn't as hard as it first seems. To fight off the problems of procrastination it helps to have your painting equipment ready set up so that you can just jump in and do it while you have the mood for it. Keep an area especially for your art work. It doesn't have to be a large space. Get into the routine of painting a small work each day. There is a great benefit in choosing to paint small works of art. These can then be finished relatively quickly in a few hours. This way you get a sense of achievement quite quickly and you can experiment with a number of new things each day. Large productions can drag on and put you off continuing. They also give a sense that they have to be finished, which means that is your central goal rather than enjoying the experience and experimenting with new ideas and techniques.

As far as materials are concerned there are no real right or wrong ones. You have to try out a range until you find ones that you like. An easel that makes you stand to paint is of great benefit in the exercise stakes but isn't needed in the artistic sense.

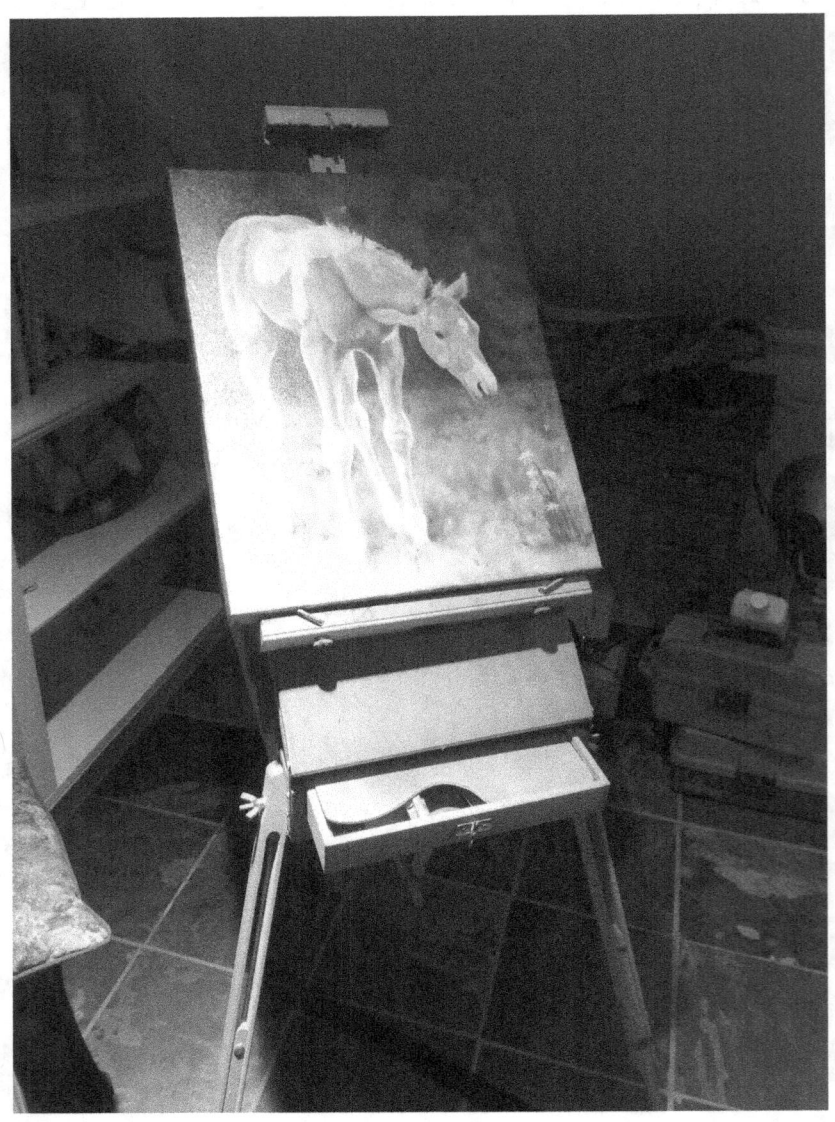

Choosing subjects to paint isn't as difficult as it might seem in that you can actually paint anything. Popular things to paint include landscapes, still life, flowers, people, vehicles, different buildings, abstract designs and animals. You can also try doing self-portraits. An easy way to decide on a still life to paint is to rove about the house looking for various objects to paint. You could then paint one or more of them. You can also have a walk about near to where you live and look for settings that look interesting. Some things might not leap out at you to start off with so it is a good idea to take lots of pictures on a digital camera. Once at home download them to a laptop so that you can study them in detail. Choose one image that has interest in the colour and composition and away you go, your next subject has been established.

This is the sort of equipment you need to start out in painting but it depends on whether you intend to do paintings in watercolour, acrylic or oil:

Watercolours

A set of watercolour tubes or cakes.

Brushes: get some Sable or Nylon ones

A pad of paper for watercolour painting

A mixing tray

Acrylic

Primary paint tubes as well as burnt umber and white

Nylon brushes

A mixing palette or tray

A range canvas boards or stretched canvas

Easel

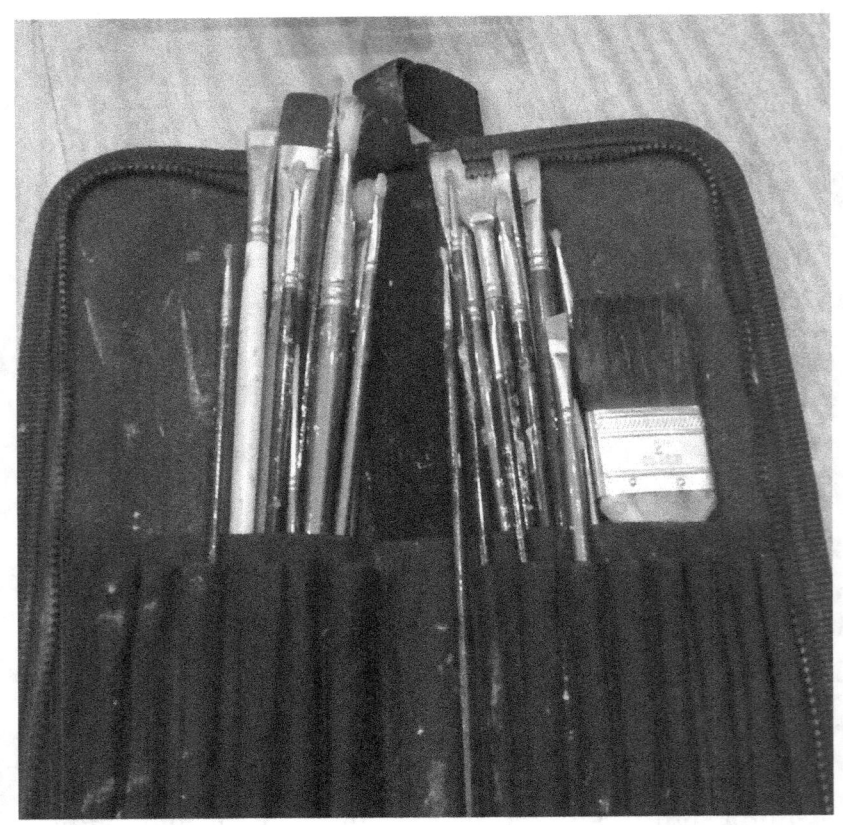

Oil

Primary paint tubes as well as Titanium white, Burnt Umber and Paynes Grey

A bottle of linseed oil

Some small jars

Brushes made from sable and bristle

A bottle of mineral spirits

Some rags

A range of canvas boards or stretched canvas

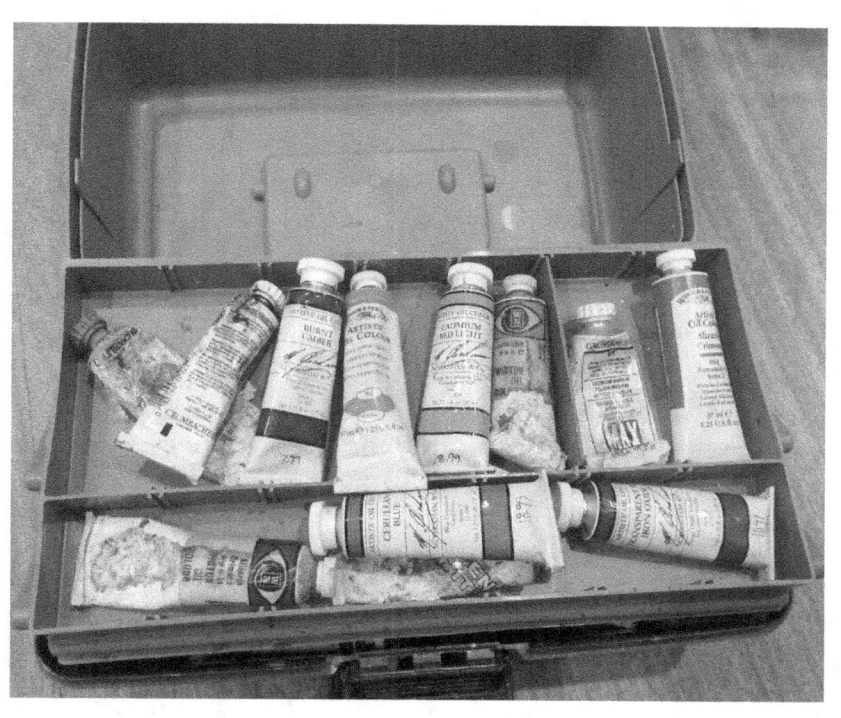

Sculpture

This isn't the most straightforward kind of art to do at home. However, to start off with you don't need all of the specialist kit such as a kiln. There are lots of ways to get going and do some modelling without all of this stuff.

You can make things simpler for yourself by choosing the right kinds of materials. Clay is ideal to start off with due to the fact that it is easy work with. So long as you keep it nice and moist you can keep on making alterations to your project as you go along. You don't need a kiln because there are lots of modelling clays that you can get that are designed to dry in the air. These types of clay are relatively cheap and therefore you can quickly get to grips with hand moulding the clay. If you don't fancy working with clay then take a look at plaster cloth wraps or even papier mache.

It is important to work out what you will be doing before you start. A good way to do this is to produce a sketch of what you are trying to create. This will then allow you to decide what kind of shapes that you need to make up the sculpture. Decide on the largest shapes that you need and then the smaller ones that will be supporting ones. Once you have done this you will be able to work out the order needed for the construction of the sculpture. This is fine for smaller shapes but if you want to make anything larger you will have to think about how it will be supported. This is typically done by making an armature which acts a bit like a skeleton for your project. The armature will not only stop your sculpture falling apart it will also allow it to be strong and light as well. Wire is a typical material used in armatures but foil and tape or even wire netting may also be used depending on the shape that you are trying to achieve. You also need to think about a base for your sculpture to be placed on. Typically this will be a piece of wood. Sculpting tools are something to invest in once you are convinced that sculpting is what you want to do. A basic set can be bought for a small amount of money. Until you get these you can improvise with other suitable items such as kitchen utensils.

When it comes to doing the work you need to make sure that surfaces are kept covered and that you have some suitable work clothes. This is especially case if you are using clay as it seems to get everywhere. You will need a jar of water to help to keep your clay moist as you work on it. Before you start make sure that you knead the clay to soften it so that it is easy to work with. As you build up your structure try to keep in mind that it will have to stand up and as a result you need to try and keep the structure balanced. Thinking about where the centre line in the sculpture is positioned can help you to balance it out when you add clay to your project. If you are using air drying clay you simply leave it to cure. After this you can glaze or paint it for greater effect.

Photography

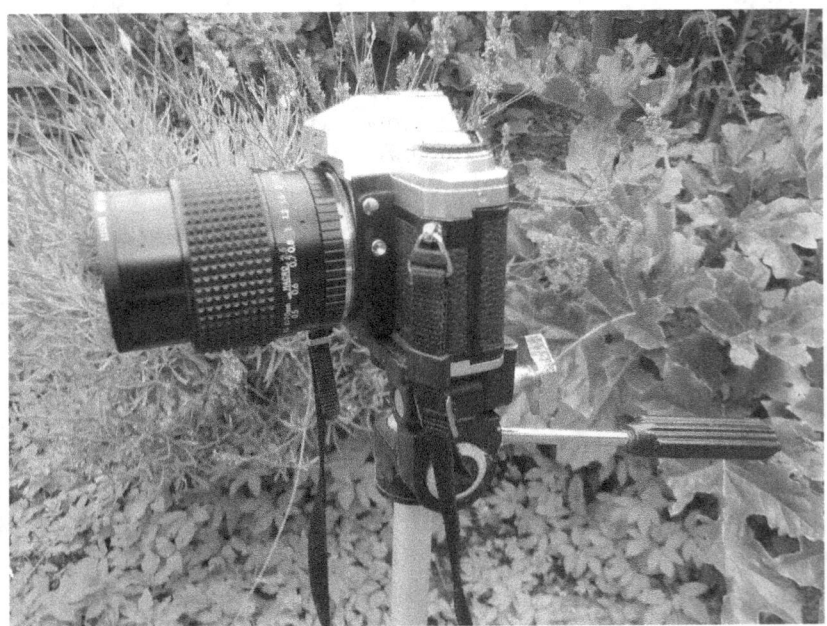

Photography is a more modern version of the visual arts but is just as valid as the other more traditional kinds of art. Anybody can take a snap with their phone, these days, but in the same way that anybody can draw something there is a lot more to doing it properly. As with other art forms there are lots of techniques to learn. At the same time, producing a good photograph requires the same kind of composition and knowledge of mixing colours as painting does. These days with digital cameras there are less barriers to taking up photography. The equipment is far cheaper than it was in the days of the chemical type of films and the results that you can get from a relatively cheap camera set up can be equally as good.

Photography can be a great hobby. Maybe you are just a bit curious about how photography works or perhaps you take a few snaps at the moment and want to develop your skills. With photography you can produce some serious art that will enthral everybody who views it. One of the miracles of photography is the ability to seize a particular moment of time and then hang on to it for keeps.

As you get into photography you will realise that you start to look at things in a different way. You will take note of different things and realise the importance of texture, light, shade and colours. Such things as buildings, trees and people will become more apparent to you. In all, you will start to see things in more detail. With the appreciation of detail comes the realisation that even ordinary things have a kind of beauty. You will notice that some colours, shades or arrangement of light will seem very pleasing and you will feel happy about it. Photography makes you more conscious of the 'here and now' because you have to take in as much as you can about the things around you, if you are to take a great picture. Distractions will melt away and you will be able to concentrate on only the one thing and that is the shot you are about to take. With all of this focus on the tasks of photography the things worrying you just won't seem that important and the general stress of life will just melt away.

Photographs are a great reminder of important things that have happened. They are fantastic pieces of art work that can be shared with family and friends. A lot of people get into photography after using it as a tool to record the life of their family members as they grow and change from one year to the next. In later years when memory issues become a problem these same photos can be used to prompt the recall of memories that may have appeared to be lost for ever.

Photography is a unique way to record the emotions of people especially in children. This in itself can have a dramatic effect on the way that you look at things. In a way, the use of a camera simplifies the ability to be creative. These days with digital cameras you can easily take many shots of the same thing altering settings and position a little each time. You can then select the most interesting photos and then subtly change them again using computer programs such as Photoshop. By changing things in this way you are letting your creative juices flow and producing your own art.

Before you get the idea that photography is just too simple to be mentally challenging, you have to realise that there is more to it than just pointing and clicking. That is just the beginning. To become proficient and produce great images is a lot more demanding. You have to learn how to use all the controls on a camera in the correct way. No more 'auto shot' images, you are now in manual adjustment territory. Besides the technical issues, there is then the artistic side of composing an image, getting the lighting right and even selecting the right moment for the best shot. The computer side of things with image processing is also an art in itself. There is one sure thing, and that is that photography certainly isn't a pass time where you will have a chance to become bored.

Taking a photograph is a very personal thing. There is no real absolutely correct way to do it. Take a bunch of photographers and tell them to photograph the same thing and the images will all end up different. That is the artistic content. You are actually sharing with others the way that you perceive the world. What you select to take photographs of, and the ways in which you embody it allows you to also display your viewpoints and judgements about the world in which we live. These expressions of your thinking will obviously change as you age and experience more of life. In short your portfolio of photographs will be a reflection of your feelings and beliefs throughout your life. This can give the people who view your photographs a great insight into what you are like as a person.

Photographs can allow you to tell a story or recount an adventure. These photographs might be in an individual form or even in a series. The way that you can use your photographs is almost endless and the decisions about what you do with your photographs will go towards the satisfaction that you receive from them. A great photograph of your adventures can be hung on a wall and become a constant reminder of good times that you have had, and as you view it, the emotions that you had at the time will flood back. This all helps to reinforce memories so that they aren't lost. In fact photos can create every kind of emotion from those that are happy to ones of great sadness and even fear. Getting your images to produce these emotions in their viewers is an important part of the skill that goes with the art of photography. In addition to this a good image can also make a person suddenly stop and think about an issue which is illustrated in the image. This can end up changing the way that people see the world. In this way your images can be very powerful indeed.

Photography doesn't lead to isolation, in fact it can help to develop your social interactions. When you are out and about taking your photos you will inevitably meet and talk to people especially if they are to become a part of the images that you are creating. If you choose to go to a photography class you will also benefit as well. Social interactions are good and you can exchange ideas about photography. Often this sort of interaction will spur you on to producing bigger and better things.

Portrait photography has its own set of important skills. The portrait needs to sum up that one person in a single image. This is the essence of a good portrait photo. This is a fantastic thing to be able to do once you have gained the necessary skills.

Unlike the other arts described in this book photography can be available to you all of the time. All you have to do is make sure that you have your camera with you. You can then catch those unique moments when they occur. Other arts require you to have a lot of equipment, a special area or a large cumbersome device to make it happen. Clearly a camera can be used just about any place and anytime.

These days a digital camera doesn't have to cost the earth. You need something where you can change the settings and has a reasonable lens. The best kind of camera has an SLR system where what you see through the view finder is actually what goes to the image sensor at the back of the camera. These tend to be more expensive but it also means that you will be able to buy a range of lenses for the camera as well. These lenses can be easily interchanged when you need them. A cheaper alternative is a bridge camera. In this case you look at an image, produced by the light that is on its way to the sensor, on a screen at the back of the camera. Good results can be obtained by this sort of camera as well. You will also need some software, on your computer, to view and adjust the images once you have taken them. Photoshop is the industry standard but there are some good free software programs, for example Gimp (http://www.gimp.org/), that can certainly do just as good a job.

Crafts

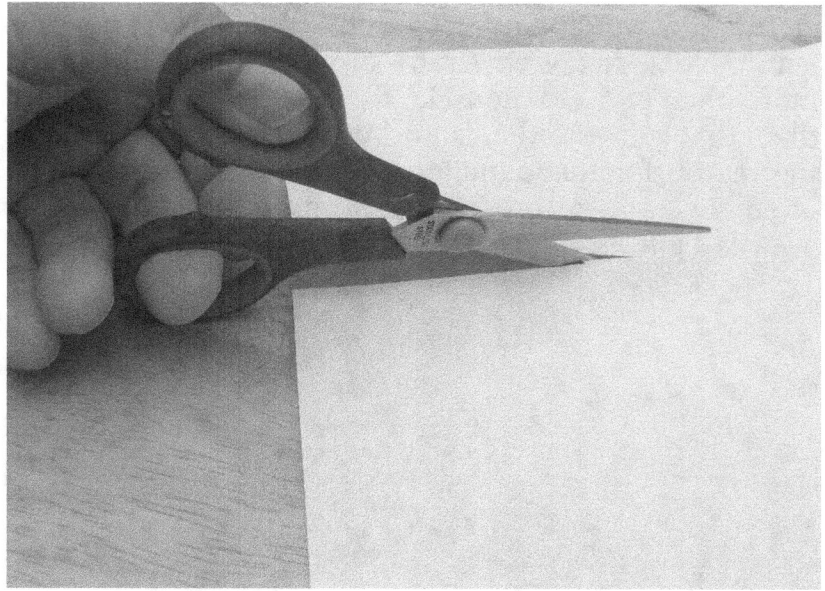

We often talk about arts and crafts as if they were one and to a certain extent there isn't a lot of difference between them. In crafts there is more of an emphasis on the fine control off the body to create interesting and practical things. Crafts give the chance to express yourself and hones hand and eye coordination and fine motor skills. While you are doing crafts stress levels become less because you can lose yourself in the work that you are doing. Once you have practised a craft skill and you get good at it you will undoubtedly get a great feeling of accomplishment. This then often leads to an increase in self-confidence and creativity which can be transferred to the rest of life outside of art. This can lead to a feeling that life has more meaning. The kinds of skills learnt by doing craft includes cutting, tracing and drawing and all this leads to the retention of better motor skills as you get older.

When doing crafts, the process of making the piece is the important thing and not necessarily the finished item. Although we all like to have that masterpiece to show off at the end we also have to think about what we have learnt along the way. Crafts are popular hobbies and more than 75% of households have somebody within them that is involved in some kind of craft hobby. Part of the reason for this popularity is that crafts are fun and often have an end product that can be used at home or even as a gift.

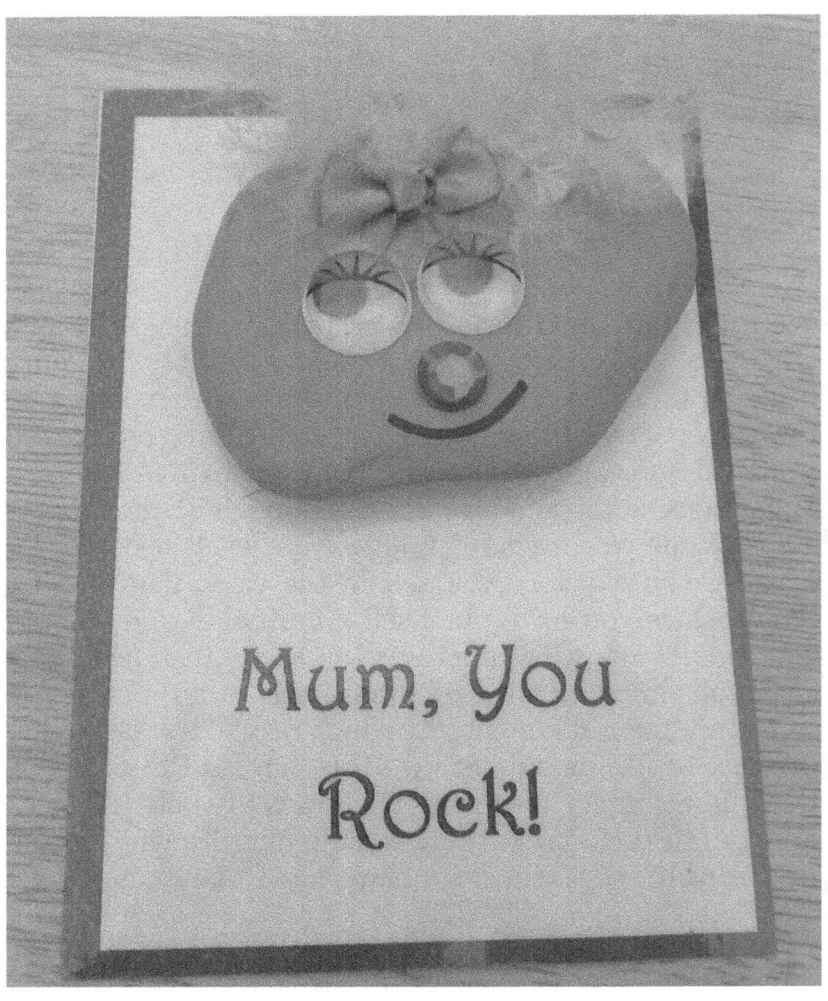

However, perhaps the most important thing is the way that doing a craft can be a distraction from the rest of the world, pacify the soul and relieve stress. Crafts are therefore good for our health, whether that be physical in nature or healing for our spirit. If you want to forget about your worries then a good craft will make sure that your mind, hands and feelings are all kept well occupied. What better distraction could there possibly be? Art and crafts have acted as a release mechanism since the beginning of man's time on the planet. Crafts are already being used with older people in care homes in the USA to try to keep minds and bodies working at the best that they can.

There have even been scientific studies into the effects of doing crafts on the human body. In one particular one from the AMA journal thirty women were selected to have their reactions to being engaged in various leisure pursuits recorded. They had their heart rate, blood pressure, skin temperature and level of perspiration measured before and after being engaged in the leisure activities. These measurements were selected because they are all good indicators of when the body is under stress. All of the activities needed the same kinds of eye and hand coordination. One of the activities was sewing and as a result, out of the women selected, half were accomplished at sewing whereas the other half were just beginners. The kinds of leisure activities used in the study included some simple sewing, painting, playing a video game, newspaper reading and taking part in a card game. Once the results of the study had been analysed it was found that sewing was rated as the most relaxing. Sewing reduced heart rate, perspiration and lowered blood pressure.

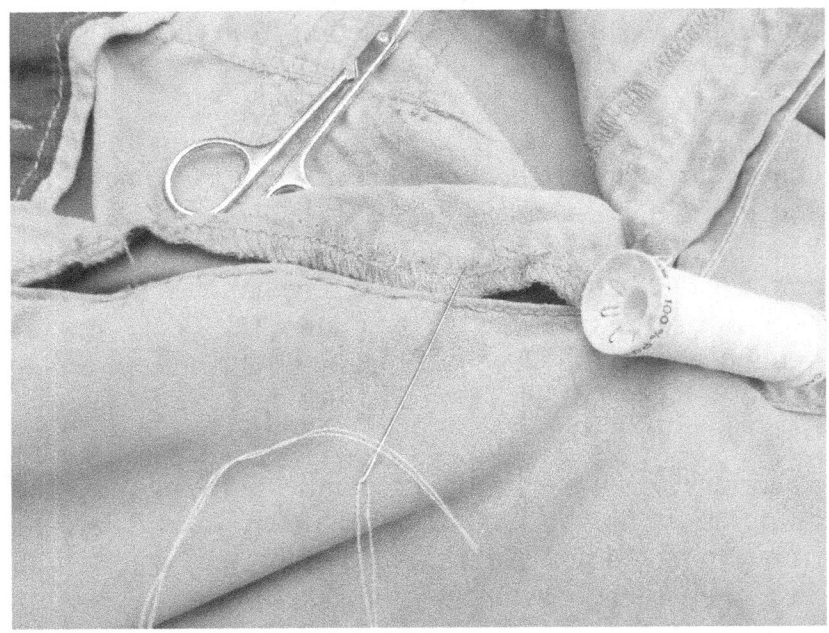

In the other activities stress levels were in fact found to be higher. In particular the highest stress levels were recorded for the tasks of playing the video game and being involved in a card game. This all backs up what craft aficionados have known all the time, and that is that being engaged in a craft diverts your attention away from workaday problems and pressures. When you are doing your craft there is no place for such things as fury, hatred, anxiety, fixations and worries. There isn't room for anything else while you are having to concentrate on what is happening in the here and now. Crafts therefore can act in a similar way to such things as meditation. It is thought that repetitive crafts such as sewing and knitting break the line of workaday thought and that it is this that frees us from the stress. This situation results in what is called a 'relaxation response' where both the body and mind become calmed. Being stress free is important for a general health and can help to lower the chances of such things as depression and heart disease. Being calm and stress free also helps the brain to work efficiently and this means that thinking and remembering things becomes easier. These are just the sorts of things that can help us to reduce the likelihood of ending up with dementia.

Despite the obvious benefits of doing crafts shown here, when it comes to real life they can come very low down on the list of things that need doing. There are so many things that impact on our everyday lives that crafts may never get a look in. As adults we are so stuck for time after working all day, dealing with domestic issues, bringing up kids and generally trying to be what everybody expects us to be. It is no wonder that there is no time to take up a craft. If you have young kids then craft can often be a part of your life because children are so open to doing them. Often they can be the ones that force you to do them just so that you can keep them happy. There can also be a sense of remorse about doing a craft because it is doing something for ourselves. We become so used to catering to everybody else's needs that doing something for yourself becomes a selfish act. We need to try and change the way that we manage our lives, and now that we know how important things like arts and crafts are to our health, we need to find the time for them. Keeping ourselves healthier as we get older needs to become a greater priority. Perhaps governments need to recognise the therapeutic value of crafts and promote them to us. After all, there will be less strain on the health service if we manage to dodge the dementia bullet. Prevention is best, especially when there is no cure!

Music as Art Therapy

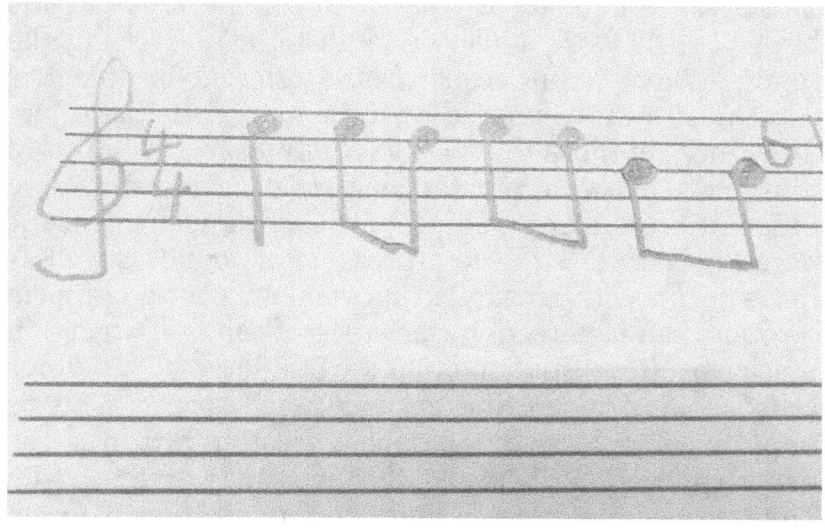

Music is another form of art that can be used to help your brain to become sharper and make your life more content and rewarding. Music can be used to good effect at all times in your life. Whereas just listening to music can help, by far the best results can be realised by actually playing music.

Like painting and drawing, music has always been a crucial factor in the development of effective culture whether it be now or in the past. It is thought that music has been a part of human culture for upwards of 60 000 years. It is interesting to note that all people respond to music in the same kinds of ways even though they may be from vastly different cultures. We all know how music can change the way that you feel. We often talk about music getting you into the right mood. This change in mood can help spark you to get on with things or can help you to concentrate on the things that you are doing.

Scientists have used neuroimaging techniques to study the effect of music on the brain. Here, the activity of the brain is shown in images where areas on the image light up when there is more brain activity in a particular part of the brain. Using these methods it has been shown that music can stimulate just about all of the areas of the brain. In this way, music is fantastic at energising the brain. When brain scans from different people are examined and compared it is found that there are differences in those that play a lot of music. The brains of musicians show a greater degree of symmetry with different areas being well proportioned. The areas of the brain associated with the processing of sound as well as those to do with controlled movement, coordination of position and direction are significantly larger in musicians. It is also found that the bundles of nerve fibres called the corpus callosum are much larger. This is important because the corpus callosum provides the nerve connections between the two sides of the brain. This means that there is more communication between these two sides of the

Brain Cross Section

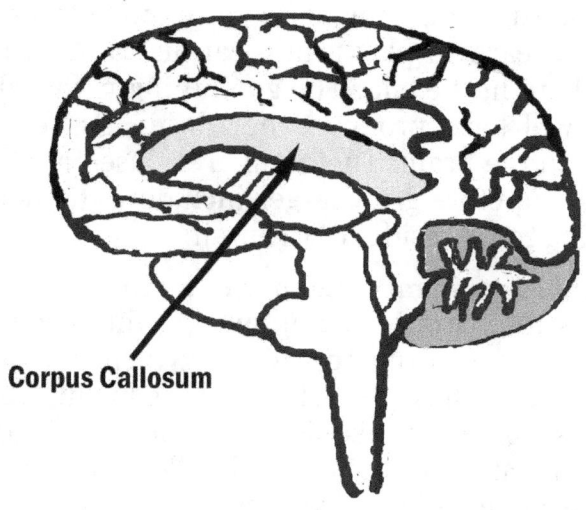

Corpus Callosum

brain in a musician. Music also causes the brain to release a substance called dopamine. Dopamine is associated with feelings of pleasure. While this in itself is good for the wellbeing of a person it has also been found to be associated with learning in the brain and the production of new and more efficient nerve pathways. Learning a musical instrument therefore causes the brain to become bigger, better and more efficient. New nervous tissue is laid down in the brain to support the new pathways being developed. Dopamine also promotes the laying down of new fatty tissue, called myelin, in the brain. Myelin causes nerve impulses to be transmitted throughout the brain more efficiently and healthy nerve cells are liberally coated with this myelin fat.

As can be seen the brain is not a static organ that is subject to a steady decline due to age. You can do things to promote the production of new brain tissue and becoming a musician is one of those things. This effect of music on the brain is not just for young people because it has been shown to be beneficial for all age groups. Although a young person's brain will develop more rapidly, because it is more pliable, an older person can also be successful at learning new things such as playing music on an instrument. It might be more difficult for an older person to learn to play a musical instrument, but they will get there in the end. The good thing is that this new learning will have produced new brain tissue and new pathways in the brain. The brain areas used a lot by musicians will therefore grow larger including the nerve band connecting the two sides of the brain.

Playing musical instruments together in a group or band has its benefits too. Group singing and playing leads to the brain releasing a hormone called oxytocin into the blood stream. This has the effect of reducing fear, increasing trust between people and bonding people together. It has also been called the 'love hormone' because it is also released after sex where it helps to bond couples together. In general this hormone will tend to make people feel happier and allow them to work well together in group situations.

Don't worry if you don't want to start along the path of learning and playing a musical instrument as you can still get value from just listening to music. Listening to music while you work can improve the work that you are doing. This is in particular the case if you have actually chosen the music that you are listening to. At work, listening to your own music is a solid path to becoming a more contented worker. It is a recognised fact that happier workers are more productive. It has been found that office workers who are allowed to listen to their own choice of music finish their work more quickly and when it comes to generating ideas and solutions to problems they are far better. Having control over what you listen to has been shown to be a key factor in improving employee outlook and output. Perhaps those teenagers who insist on listening to music while they do their school or college homework have been right all along!

Music's influence on a person's mood is well known and science has gone a long way to show that listening to cheery music can put somebody into a good mood. Stress can often lead to depressive situations and listening to upbeat music can help with this because it leads to a reduction in the hormone cortisol which is associated with stress. Happy music can give you feelings of hope and a sense that you are in control of your own destiny. These optimistic feelings are of benefit to the whole of the body. Sad music can also be helpful in the right situations. When times are bad listening to sad music can be soul cleansing. It can help you to deal with all of the emotions that you are going through.

Dementia leads to the breakdown of brain tissues and with this breakdown go the memories and coordination abilities of a person. It stands to reason therefore that the more healthy brain tissue that there is in the brain the longer it will take for a significant amount to be lost due to the disease. Therefore, if you can build up the amount of brain tissue that you have before these conditions take a hold the longer you can hang on to your mental capabilities. Music and art in general is therefore an important way for people to increase their healthy brain mass. Do it before you get old and the longer you will remain healthy and lucid. It doesn't matter when you start as learning a musical instrument can benefit you at any age. In fact right now is a good time to start your own musical project!

It has been found that even people with the dementia condition can benefit from listening to music. This is especially the case if the music is from their past. Certain music is often associated with particular things that happened to a person in the past. When a person hears that music again it can dredge up memories from their past that it was assumed were lost forever. It might be the song that was played at their wedding or on a particularly happy event such as a birthday or graduation from college or university. This works rather like the situation when you smell something and you say that it took you right back to being in your mother's kitchen or in the home garden on a summer night. Keep listening to music now and watch those memories come flooding back.

Even with severe cases of dementia music can be seen to have an effect on individuals. When they hear music that they know from their past you can see the recognition on their faces. Beams of happiness will spread across them and even though they can't communicate verbally you will know that it has hit the spot.

Getting Started
with Music

The majority of people enjoy listening to music. We have music on in the car while we drive, music on our iPods and phones while we travel on public transport or walk about, music on the stereo system in the house. Music is often on in places that we visit whether it be a pub or restaurant. All visual media comes over better with a music track too. Without the music a film would seem kind of sterile and uninteresting. Even listening to all of this music has a benefit in that it stimulates our senses and our brains respond to the changes in mood, tempo and tone. We have a built in appreciation of music and most of us know what we like. If you remember back in time to being a teenager I am sure that you will realise how important music was for us. It wasn't just that particular decade of being a teenager it just seems that the mind is more open to music then. It is probably something to do with all the hormones surging around the body at that time in a person's life. The funny thing is that the music we listen to at this important part of our lives sticks with us. We always say that it was the best music ever and this is partly why older people pour scorn on the modern teenager and their musical tastes. It just isn't how music is supposed to be like. As a result, if you are stuck and wondering what music to focus on just get the old albums out and have a listen. It will all come flooding back including all of the emotions that went with it. What about if you could play this music or sing it? That would be good too eh? Having found the type of music that you resonate with you need to work out what to do. Think about what you like the most, Was it the singing, guitar playing, keyboards or maybe the stunning saxophone solo? Perhaps you could take up one of these instruments or do some singing?

Singing

The voice is really another musical instrument but it is a part of your body too. As with all musical instruments some people are naturals at singing but the rest of us have to work at it. If you were a natural when it comes to singing it is likely that you would already be involved with it now or at some time in the past. The rest of us need some encouragement. If you are interested in taking up singing and haven't done much about it then you should seriously consider having lessons. One of the main reasons for this is that if you don't sing using good technique you can seriously damage your vocal cords and in turn your voice. You have to learn the basics before you can progress. Having said this, a lot of people do just get on with their singing and do ok in the end.

On the whole, singing is something that you do with others. You can sing solo, and some folk singers make a career of just doing that. I know some people who will turn up at a folk night and sing a few songs on their own and go down really well. However, if you are just taking up singing you will probably be thinking of joining a choir or singing as part of a group with other musicians playing backing instruments. You don't even have to be the main singer. You can be a backing singer for a main artist. Playing your part in a group is beneficial to the brain because of the coordination skills that you have to apply to working with others. You will also benefit from all of the social interactions that take place.

You can get DIY books and audio/video recordings as courses in order to help you improve your singing. In the end though, there is nothing better than getting out there and rehearing with a band, doing some gigs and producing some recordings.

Playing a Musical Instrument

Not all musical instruments are created equal. In this, I mean that some are easier to get a tune out of compared to others. The easiest instrument to use in order to play a tune is a keyboard. You put your finger on a key and a note comes out. Compare this with a flute and you could easily find that getting your mouth into the right position to sound a note from the flute head piece could take a week or more. It is all about technique. The same thing applies to the guitar. Fretting a note takes some skills that your fingers have to learn and this takes time. This doesn't mean to say that a keyboard doesn't have complex issues.

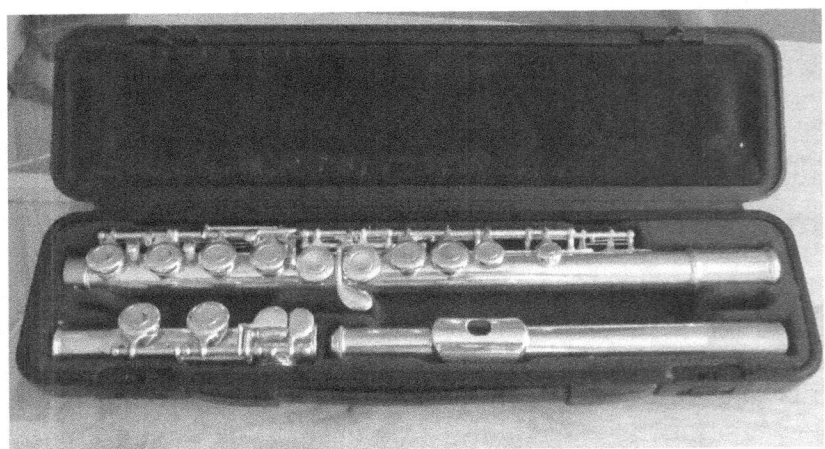

On a flute you only have to play one note at a time. On a keyboard you could be playing three different parts at the same time with multiple notes. This would be a bass line, a chord and a melody. Instruments are as difficult to play as you make them. To play any instrument to its full potential takes a lot of skill, practice and time. Remember it is the complex nature of playing any musical instrument that is going to give your brain the mental workout that it needs.

A lot of people take up the guitar because it is a very popular instrument in bands of all kinds. You have to think about what you want to do with the guitar in the end. You can play tunes on a guitar or chords as part of a rhythm unit in a band. A lot of people want to play the lead solo type of guitar because it is what makes guitar heroes. This sort of playing only comes off if you are part of a band. This is not a bad thing, because of all of the social interaction and the coordination it needs to get a group of musicians to work together in sync. The quickest way to get some love back from a guitar is to use it to play chords as a backing while you sing a song. This isn't as hard as it sounds. You don't even have to be able to sing very well in order to get quick rewards in completed songs by using your guitar in this way. So, what is really important is to think about what you expect to get from playing your instrument. Choosing wisely will mean that you will continue to play your instrument for many years to come. Choose unwisely and the instrument won't get played and will end up as shelf ware at the back of your wardrobe.

Having lessons to play your musical instrument is a good idea. You will progress more quickly and therefore get more enjoyment as well as the social aspect of having to go to the lesson itself. Lessons maybe individually or in groups. In an individual lesson you will get the benefit of more attention of the teacher. In a group situation you have to share the teacher but you get social benefit with other learners as well as being able to gauge your progress against the other students. The teacher will also give you work to practice which will be an incentive to practice the instrument. This is important because learning through practice is the bit that grows your brain, improves the connections between the different areas of the brain and develops your motor skills. Using a music stand for your practice pieces of music allows you to stand while you play your instrument. This of course is adding a form of physical exercise to your music sessions. In general we sit for too long during the day so a music stand is a good way to make sure that you stand for some of it.

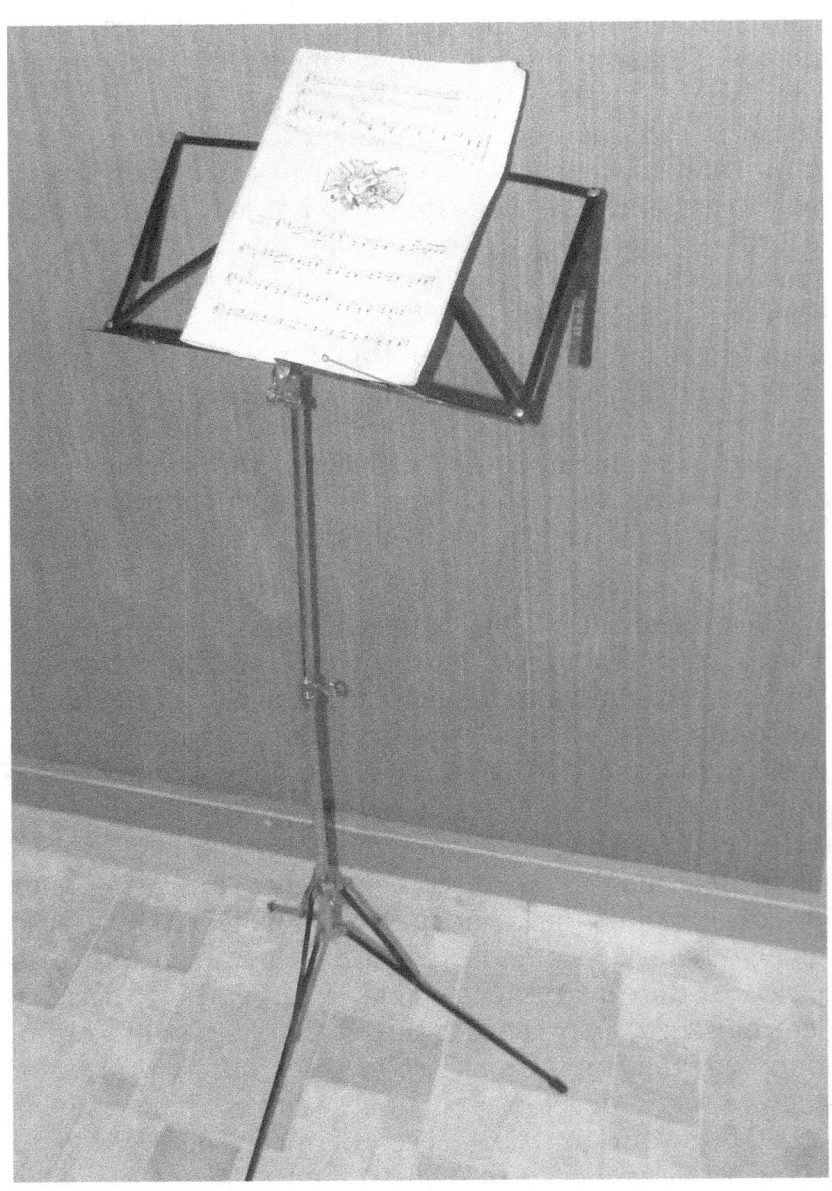

On a guitar the motor skills learnt concerns the ability of the brain to put the fingers on the right fret at the right time to sound the correct musical note. Some guitarists call this your 'finger memory' although it is your brain and its coordination with the muscles in your arm that actually do this.

There are plenty of DIY books, audio tapes, video DVDs and online lessons that you can access in order to teach yourself how to play the instrument of your choice. If you do go the DIY route it works even better if you know a friend who already plays the same instrument. You can then ask them for help and tips as you progress in learning the instrument. When I started learning guitar I had a friend who was a couple of years older than me and I used to go round each weekend and pick his brains about various techniques and instrument problems. At the same time I had a few different books on how to play. Between the two things I managed to start playing reasonably well. I then joined a group and even went out and played gigs. Once you learn a musical instrument you don't forget it. As they say it is 'like riding a bike'. You may get a little rusty over the years, if you stop playing, but the ability is always there. If you used to play an instrument in the past but have let it slide for a few years take it up again, join a band, why not?

The Art of Language

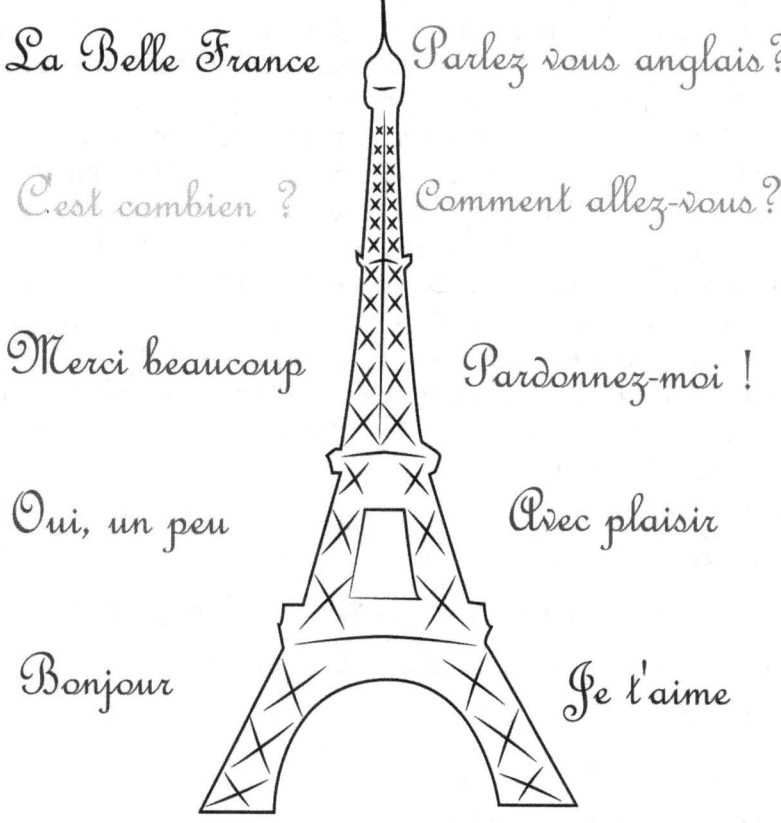

La Belle France

C'est combien ?

Merci beaucoup

Oui, un peu

Bonjour

Parlez vous anglais ?

Comment allez-vous ?

Pardonnez-moi !

Avec plaisir

Je t'aime

Whether you consider languages as a form of art or not doesn't really matter. It can be considered to be at the centre of human creativity and it is what separates us from other animals including our nearest ape relatives.

The advent of language is thought to be responsible for the original burst in creativity that the human race produced way back in time. As it is related to art it is no surprise that learning a language stimulates similar areas of the brain to other art forms. It has been shown that learning another language besides your natural one leads to enhancements in concentration, memory and even brainpower. It is therefore no wonder that learning a second language is thought to decrease the risk of suffering from dementia type illnesses.

Dealing with language is just about the most difficult thing that the human brain has to do. Due to the complicated nature of languages, dealing with a second one makes the brain have to work very hard. The more effort that is used the greater the benefits for brain health. The harder that your brain works the stronger that it gets. By learning a new language and using it you can keep your brain active and hedge against the aging process. It doesn't matter what age you are as you are never too old to take up a new language. By learning and using a new language you can improve your cognitive abilities and general workings of your brain. The more languages that you learn the more enhanced the brain functions become.

Being Bilingual or multilingual can give improvements in:

Mathematics, reading, knowledge and use of words

General thinking, acumen and brain power

Awareness of surroundings

Ability to focus on things

Recalling lists and orders of things

Making decisions

Forward planning

Multitasking

Remembering things

working memory

Adaptability to change

Flexible thinking

Imagination, ingenuity and creativity

Ability to actively listen

On the physical side a second language leads to the brain becoming larger and better connections being established between the different areas of the brain. In particular there will be an increase in the size of the brain's language centre as well as the hippocampus which is tasked with putting together, storing and recalling memories. This increase in size of the hippocampus has been observed in studies by scientists in Sweden. They used MRI scans on the brains of people before and after they had started learning a new language. MRI scans have been used in other studies to determine how connections in the brain change while learning a new language. In this case people who spoke English had brain scans during the time they were trying to learn different words in a Chinese language. The MRI scans revealed that new nerve connections had been made across the various regions of the brain. These changes reflected the changes needed in the way the brain had to work while learning the new language. The changes in the brain's organisation could be seen to take place in even just a few weeks after starting to learn the Chinese words. Neither were the changes restricted to young people. It was found that even older people's brains responded in a similar way. Previously, scientists had concluded that the brain's ability to develop was restricted to young people while the body is growing. This new evidence gives hope to the older generation in that it appears that the brain can grow and mould to new situations never mind how old that you are.

What everybody wants is protection against the effects of aging and the avoidance of brain conditions such as dementia and Alzheimer's. Currently doctors prescribe drugs to try and delay the onset of dementia. These drugs only work to postpone the creep of dementia for up to a year. After this time you still end up suffering the condition. This happened to my mother and the drugs also had side effects which weren't very pleasant either. How much better to do some language work before the aging process takes hold and protect yourself against the onset of dementia. This is where learning a language is such a good proposition. There are no nasty side effects and no horrible drugs to take. In comparison to drugs it is estimated that learning another language can put off the onset of dementia for up to about 5 years. As you can see this is a far better result than using the drugs. In the case of my mother I didn't really notice any substantial effects of the drugs she was given and she had a bad reaction with at least one of the prescribed drugs.

In the case of older people, brain scans have been used to try and determine the changes that take place on learning a new language. Those ones who were bilingual had greater brain activity when compared to those who only knew their own native language. It was also noted that their brains were working in a more efficient way and in this respect they were acting like the brain of a much younger person. These increases in brain power and the plasticity of the older brain have been put down to the fact that they actually have some brain power built in as a reserve. It is thought that this reserve is actually there to offset the normal aging of the brain and is nature's way of trying to keep us sharp as we get older.

If you are bilingual there is evidence to suggest that learning yet another language will give you even greater benefits when it comes to the aging process. As a result it is in your interest to keep on learning different languages rather than just sticking at being bilingual. It has been noted that multilingual children benefit from their unique situation in that they often do better in tests and have greater academic achievement in school. Languages learnt while you are young give benefits that last a lifetime and will still act to keep you sharp during your old age. As a result it doesn't really seem to matter when you learnt your second or third language.

On the other side of things it is never too late to actually learn a new language. As well as this, if you already know a second language then actually using it helps to increase the sharpness of the brain. Learning yet another language will cause further boosts in brain power. As an older individual you may feel that starting on a new language is too daunting to even consider. You may be also be wondering if it is even worth bothering to do. The good news here is that you don't have to become fluent in it to get benefits. Just starting along the route of learning the language and gaining some ability in it can have an effect on the brain. You can even start by just building up a basic vocabulary by learning a few words in the new language each day. It has been shown that you don't need to know that many words in a language to actually do some communicating. If you learn one hundred of the most common words then you will have a knowledge of half of the words used in daily conversations. This means that with a little guesswork you will be able to actually communicate with somebody in a meaningful way. There are even lessons that are designed to get you to your 100 words and details of these can be found by searching on the internet. These lessons are also often free which is another bonus. With just a small number of words each day it would only take a few months to get to the one hundred target. However, there is no need to stop there. Learn some more words and you will be communicating

71

even better. Even at this basic rate of learning you could be reading the language in just about a year.

The reason that languages are so good at stimulating the brain is because it gives the brain something to work on that is both complicated and out of the normal day to day things that it has to deal with. Your brain loves this kind of thing. A lot of people resort to brain training games or things like crosswords and other puzzles to do a similar thing. Languages offer much more than a game or puzzle can in that they have practical applications in the world. It is not games for just gaming sake. In this way it is a much more fruitful way to entertain yourself. You shouldn't forget the cultural additions that go with a language either. With a new language under your belt the travel opportunities just shout out at you. Getting to use your new language gets you to meet new people who will also stimulate your brain with their different views and cultures. All this communication with fellow human beings will give a sense of satisfaction and confidence as well as being enjoyable. Indeed, learning a new language can open up a whole new world of opportunities which are bound to get you thinking, and thinking is the key because the brain thrives on it.

Conclusion

Now is the time to start thinking about what you are going to do to try and put off the possibility of suffering from dementia when you get older. You might not be able to stop it affecting you eventually, but putting it off a few years has got to be worth it.

Obviously there are lots of factors to consider when it comes to preventing dementia, from diet and exercise through to smoking, alcohol consumption and keeping your mind active. As we have seen in this book keeping your mind active is one of the most important things that you can do. If you can combine that with exercise all the better.

There are a lot of ways to keep your mind active but the more pleasurable the activity is, the greater the benefits to the brain. The arts are a fantastic way to give your brain a workout. Avoiding the routine and dealing with complex meaningful problems is the best. Art ticks all the boxes and all you have to do is put aside some time to do it.

The more art activities that you do the better. There is no reason why you can't do a range of things. Pick an art activity such as painting and combine it with learning a musical instrument and a new language. All these are pleasurable things to do. All you have to do is find the time. It doesn't have to take up all of your time, and besides as we get older a lot of us find that we have time on our hands a plenty. When it comes to retirement don't just spend your time in front of the TV. That is a sure-fire route to 'Brain death' if ever there was one! As a person who has retired relatively recently I always try to keep busy. A walk each day is one thing that I try to do. 6000 steps a day keeps the joints and circulatory system ticking over nicely. That's a minimum. I try to walk more if I can. Each route I take has a café to visit as a reward. We all need rewards! While at the café I read the next chapter of a book on my Kindle. Currently I am reading the complete works of Jules Verne but 'Game of Thrones' is my favourite book series. I have my guitar on the seat next to me so that I can pick it up whenever I have the mind to.

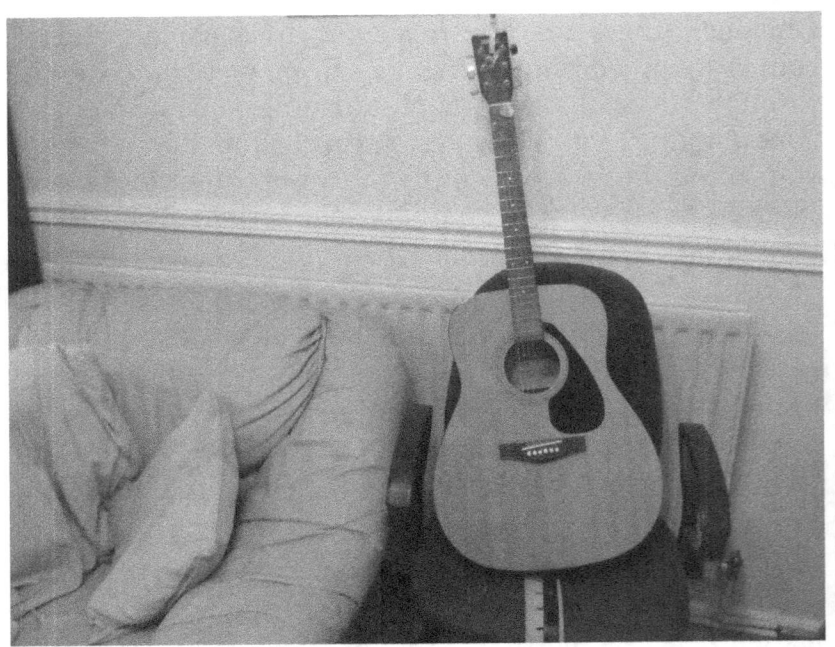

Guitar at the ready

If I am watching TV I listen to some of the tunes that come up and then pick up my guitar and try and play them. Other times I try to write and record some songs. I have a mini studio for this setup in the garage ready to go whenever I need it. It takes up a minimum amount of space and only cost me a few hundred dollars to put together.

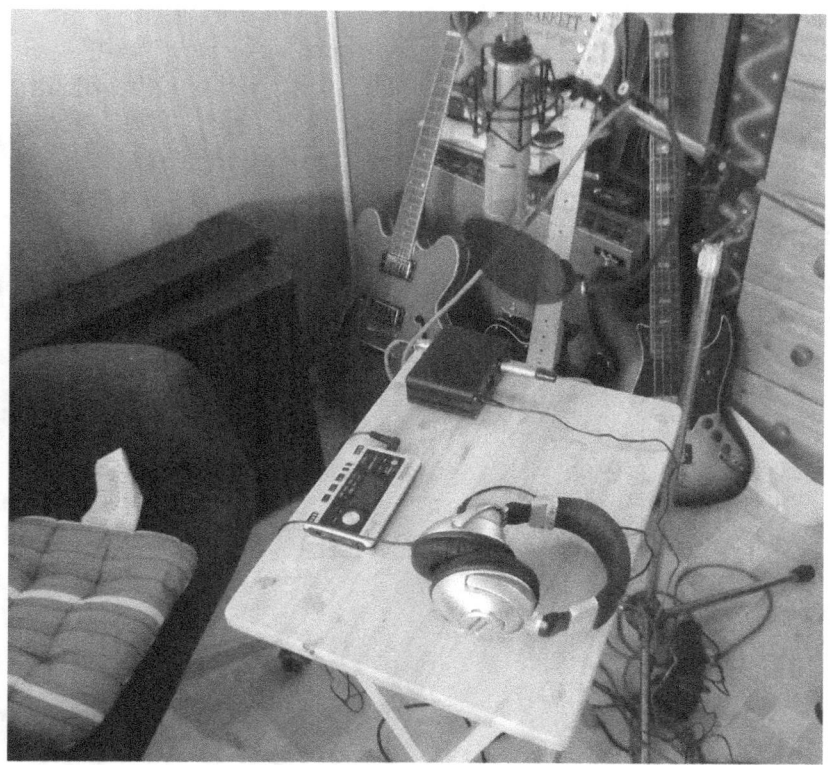

Corner of the garage for a studio

I have other musical instruments around the house which also can be played: such as a mandolin, bass guitar and a keyboard too. In the past I have studied languages and have some French and a holiday amount of Turkish to keep me going when I visit there. Currently I am trying to learn the language 'Twi' for a visit to relatives in Ghana in a few months' time. Although I have some books for this, I recently found a complete course for this language on the internet which was absolutely free. As you can see there are lots of different art related tasks that you can do piece meal during a day. It all just flows together. Obviously, if you have to fit work into your day as well, then time can be more limiting. However, watch a little less TV and you will quickly see those extra hours build up. Don't try to do too many things if you have restricted time. Concentrate on one form of art and aim to do it well. Maybe you always wanted to play guitar? Well now is the time to do it. Get yourself a cheap instrument and book a half hour lesson every week or two. The lessons will give you the incentive to keep going and pretty soon you will be playing that guitar, buying extra instruments and after a while your house will be filled with music too!

The main thing to learn from this book is that it is never too late to take up an art form. The sooner that you do, the sooner that your brain will start to reap the benefits. Work your brain hard and make it grow some new nerve cells and a greater number of nervous connections. If you don't do this now you probably won't remember, in the future, what it was that you were supposed to do in the first place. Good luck and may your art be with you!

About The Author

Tim Vincent is a retired biologist who was involved in education for a number of years. He still maintains his scientific interests and has a blog on nutrition and diet related issues (http://medicinalplantsinformation.com). He also enjoys creating picture books for children. He also has an interest in music and runs a guitar related web site(http://www.settingupaguitar.co.uk). This book is a true cross over between his interests in science and the arts and Tim believes that Art really does have a role to play in keeping us fit and healthy into old age.